Dowdy Dot to Glamorous Gail
by Sabina Saturn

Anyone can look plain or glamorous. It's a choice.
Many famous beauties have been "plain Janes".

Even Princess Grace, Princess Diana could look frumpy.
This book explores how they evolved into beauties with
style and how you can too.

Table of Contents

Princess Grace - a Plain Jane?

Princess Grace could be a "plain Jane? Yes.

In her role in the 1954 film "Country Girl", Grace Kelly was made to look plain, with little make-up, and drab clothing.

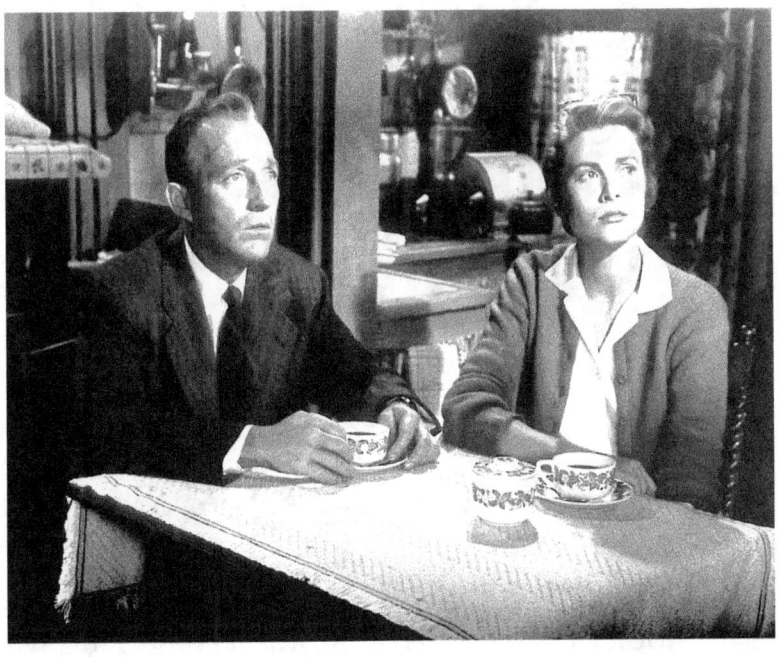

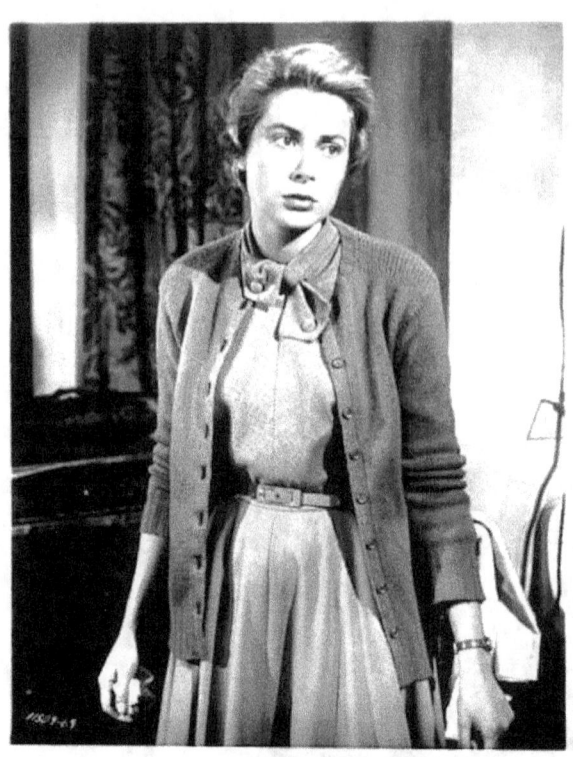

She certainly would not attract attention, looked drab and plain.

However, look at Grace Kelly at her first meeting with Prince Rainier:

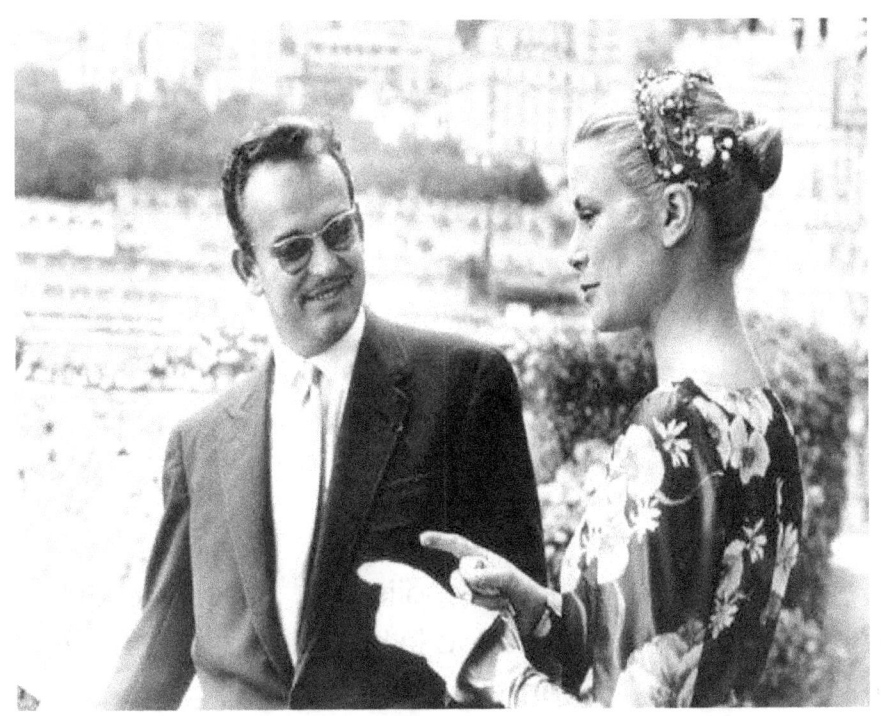

He didn't stand a chance.

All the World is a Stage

Clothes are important. They are a kind of language, conveying what you think of yourself. They give messages, especially to men. Stage directors recognize the value of costumes on stage in the theatre.

You can wear drab clothing, pay little attention to style and fashion or make-up, remain overweight. Or you can make another choice.

Look at these words that describe unfashionable:
bedraggled   messy   sloppy   slovenly   tacky
tattered   threadbare   dowdy   drab   dull   inelegant
worn   old-fashioned   plain   rough   unfashionable
ungroomed   unstylish   unpolished

Look at the words for "stylish":
beautiful   chic   classy   polished   sleek   smart
snazzy   trendy   dressed to kill   dressed to the teeth
in vogue   sassy   sharp

Princess Grace learned how to present herself with grace
and poise. She knew how to enhance her beauty with
style.

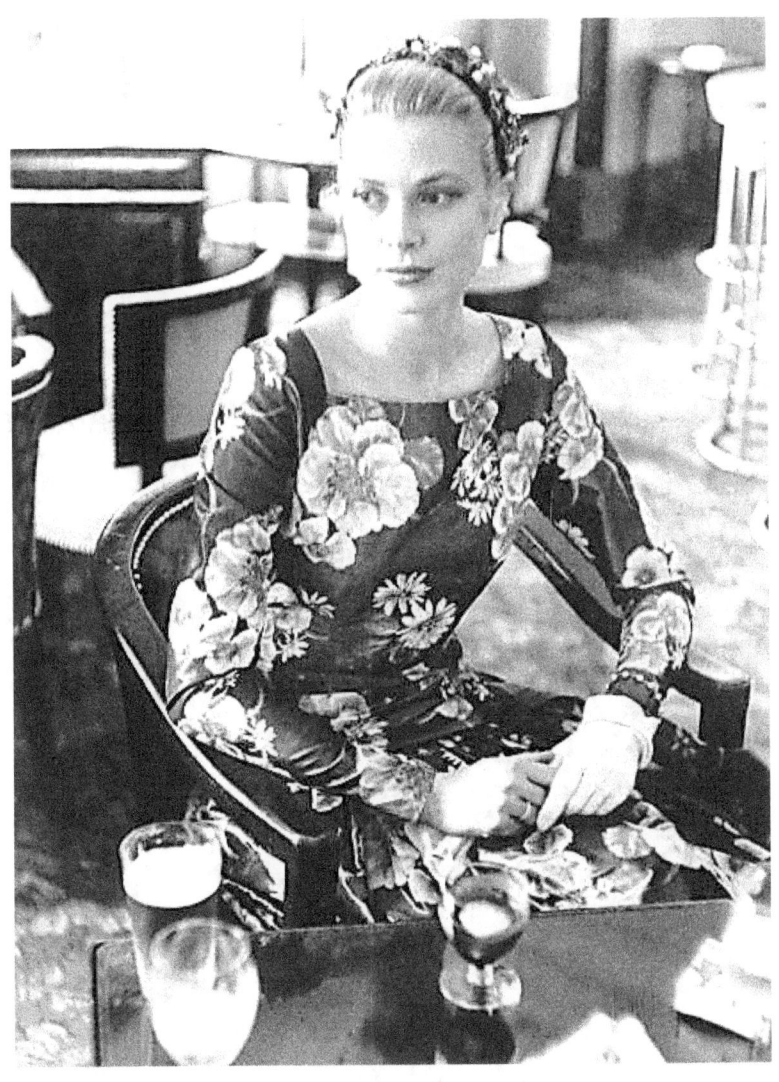

The story is that when Princess Grace first met Prince Rainier of Monaco, her hotel had lost electricity and she couldn't dry her hair properly, so put it up. Her dresses were not ironed and wrinkled. She had originally planned to wear another dress. She was reluctant to go, but she went.

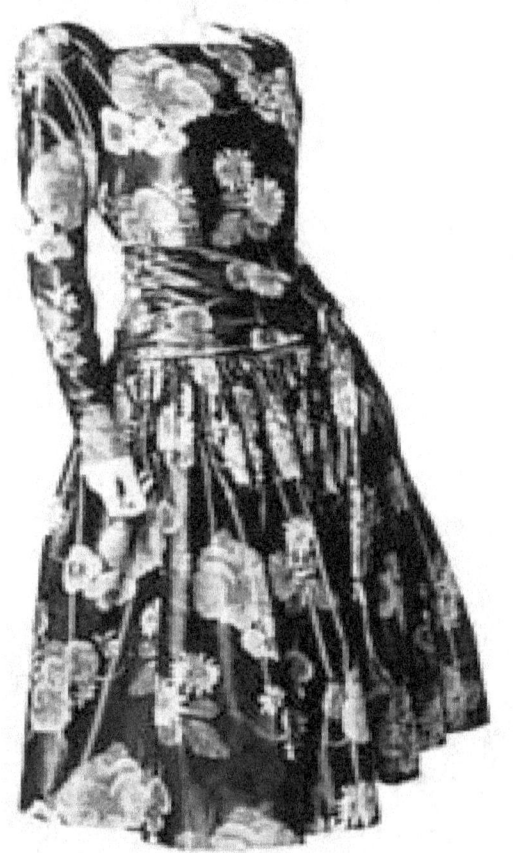

She selected a stunning dress.

It is obvious some thought was put into her attire and appearance that day.

"Simplicity is the keynote of all true elegance."
~ Coco Chanel

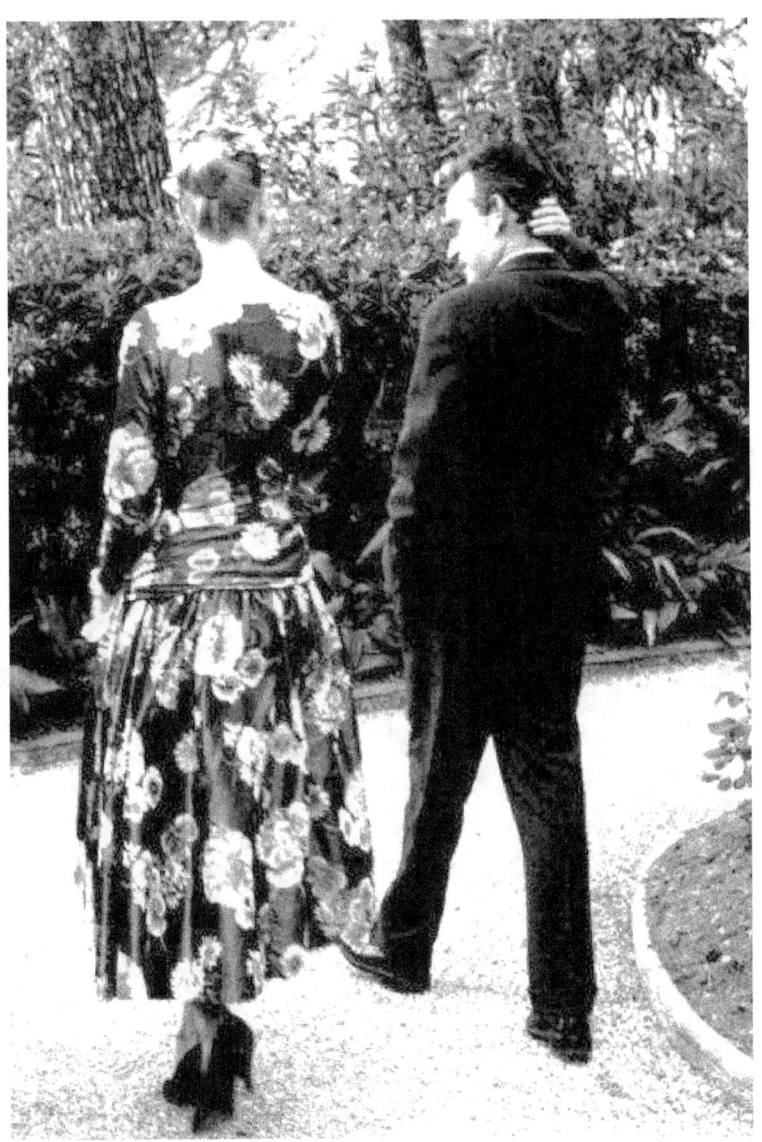

I love the dress Grace Kelly wore for her civil wedding ceremony. It was a creamy lacy perfection:

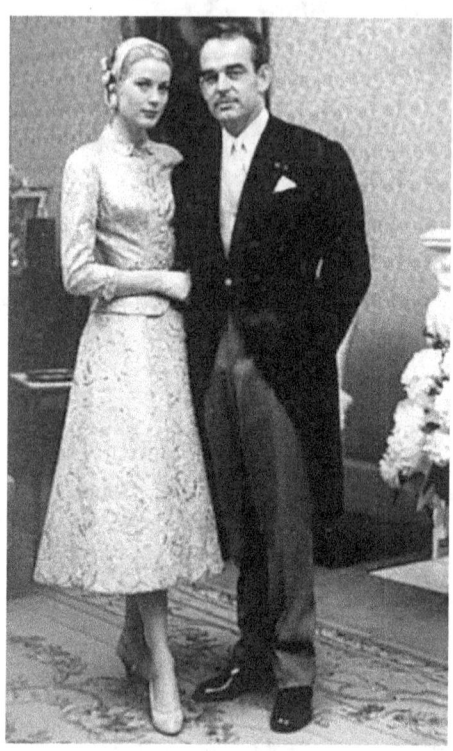 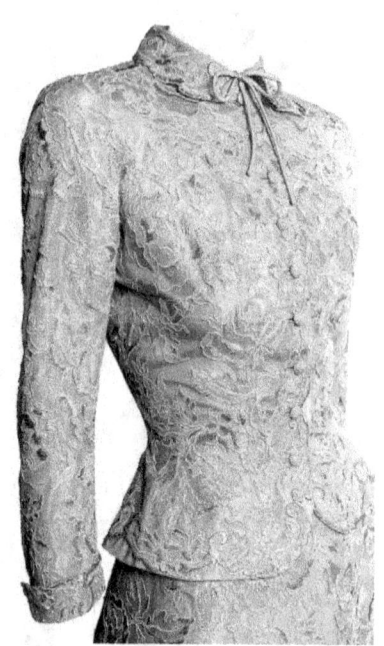

Grace Kelly's civil wedding service suit, 1956, designed by Helen Rose of MGM Studios

These clothes were the epitome of the understated, elegant Grace Kelly from her Hollywood days.

Grace studied ballet while she was young. Ballet left it's mark on Grace - lithe figure and limbs, and perfect posture. Grace stated that she stayed in shape by walking for at least an hour a day - and very quickly.

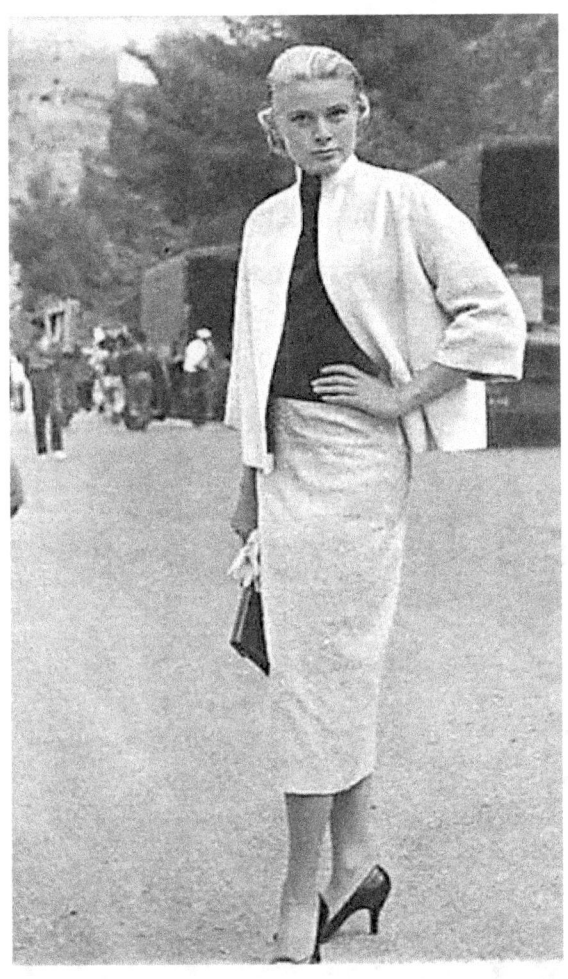

When asked if she dieted, Grace said: "I try to avoid that as much as possible. A crash diet would make me nervous and bad-tempered," she continued. "I do enjoy good food but try to eat correctly, the right things. I am aware of the importance of having well-balanced meals. We have whole-meal bread and whole rice, and I tend to avoid sugar."

Grace knew style and how to use it. She had dated Oleg Cassini, a renowned fashion designer. Her style wasn't overdone. Just right.

"Sweatpants are a sign of defeat.
You lost control of your life
so you bought some sweatpants."
~ Karl Lagerfeld

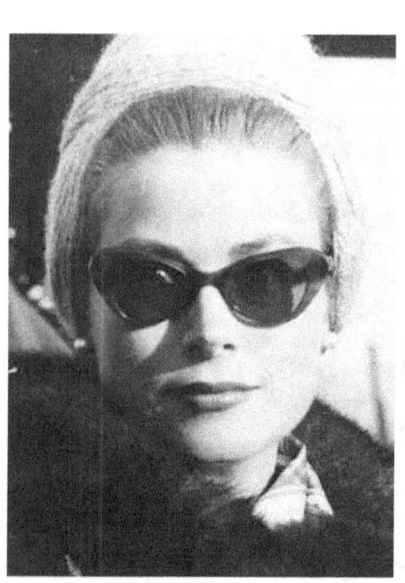 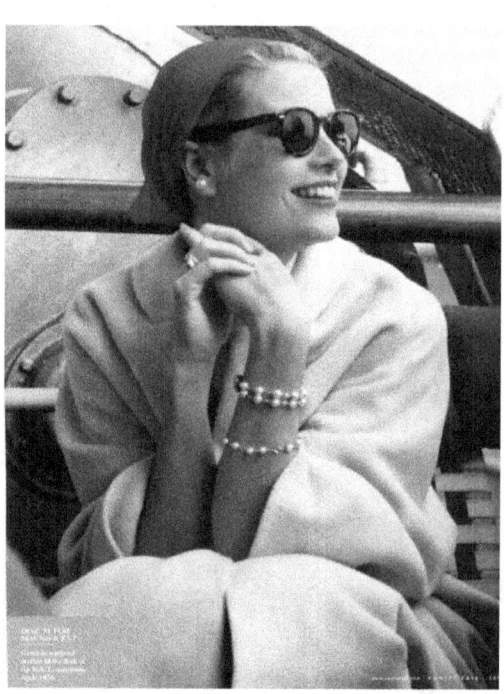

Grace's sunglasses, the cat-eye style,
perfectly counterbalanced her square jaw-line.

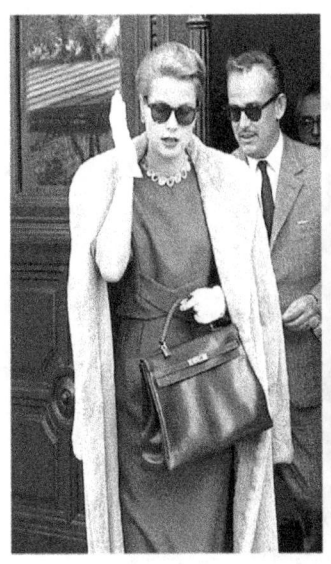 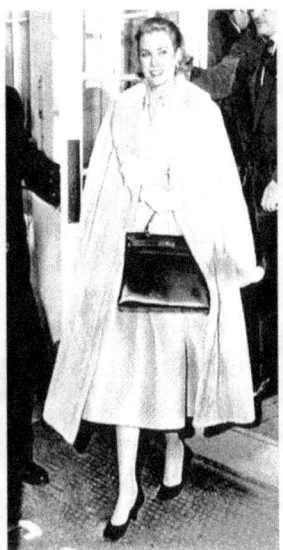 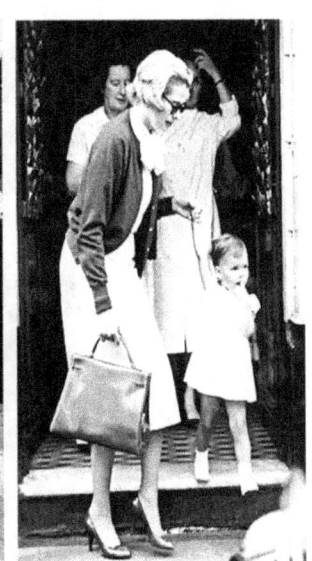

Grace used a large handbag to divert the eye during her pregnancies. A Hermes bag was even created in her honor.
Perfect style:

"Simplicity is the keynote of all true elegance."
~ Coco Chanel

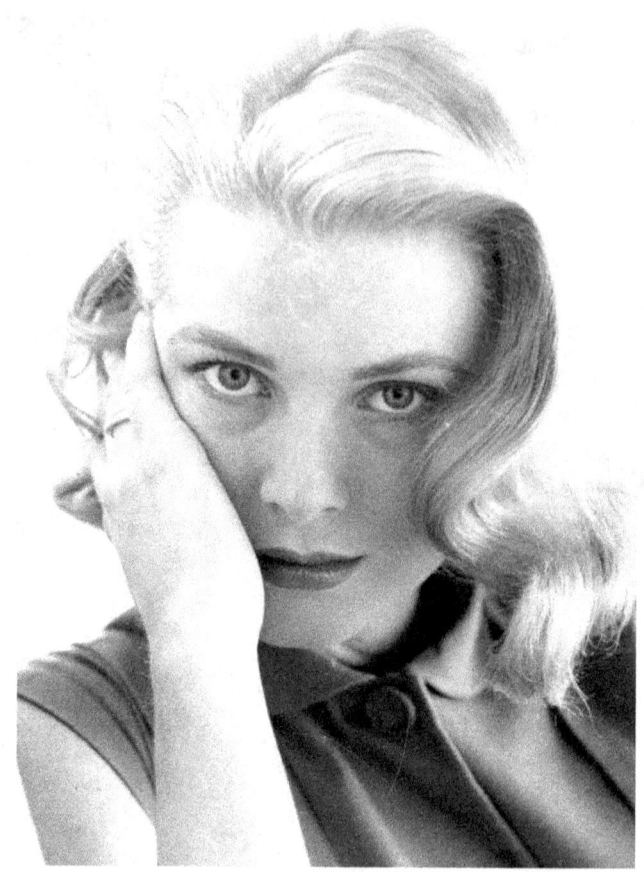

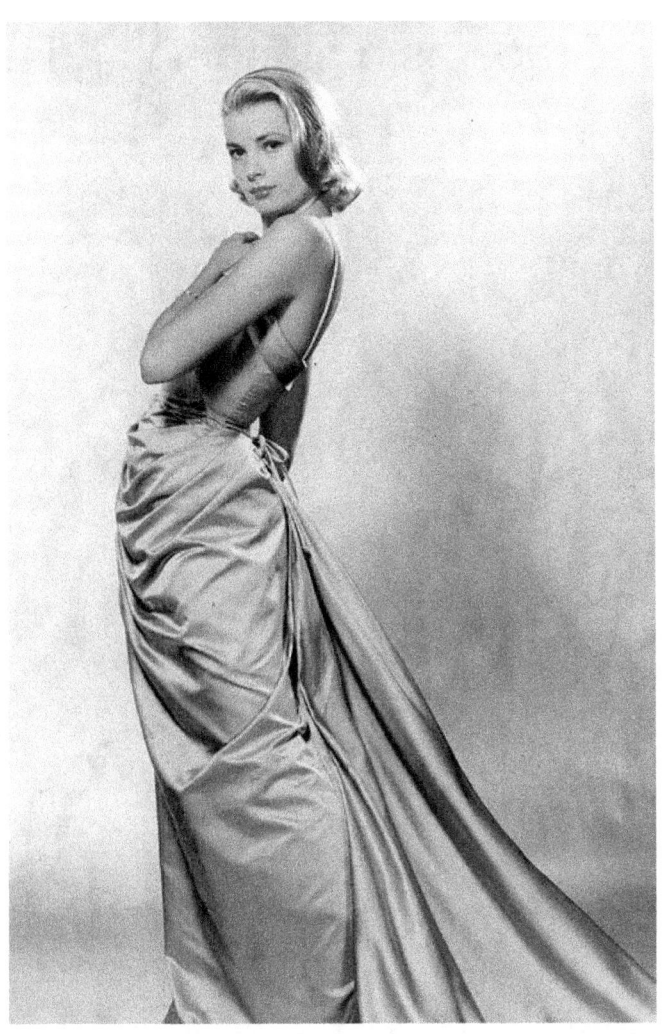

Grace as a stunning bride:

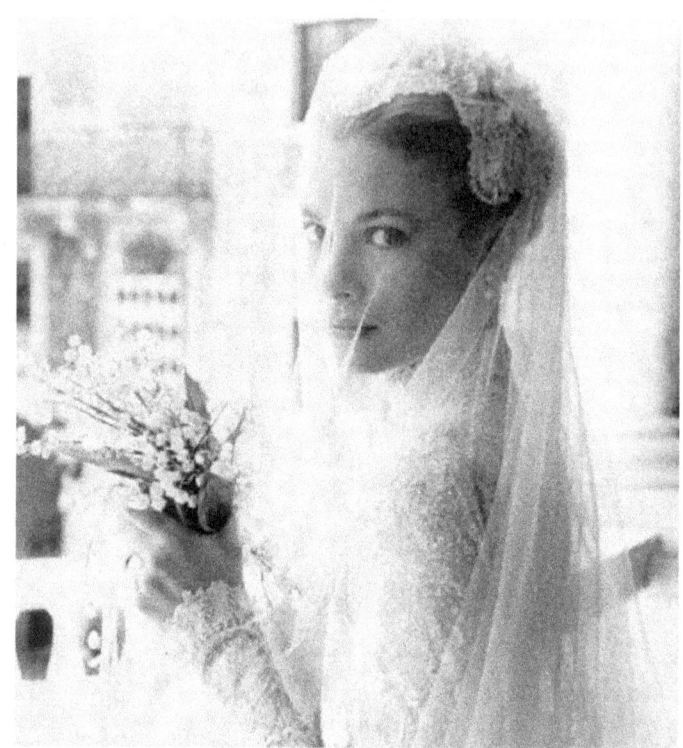

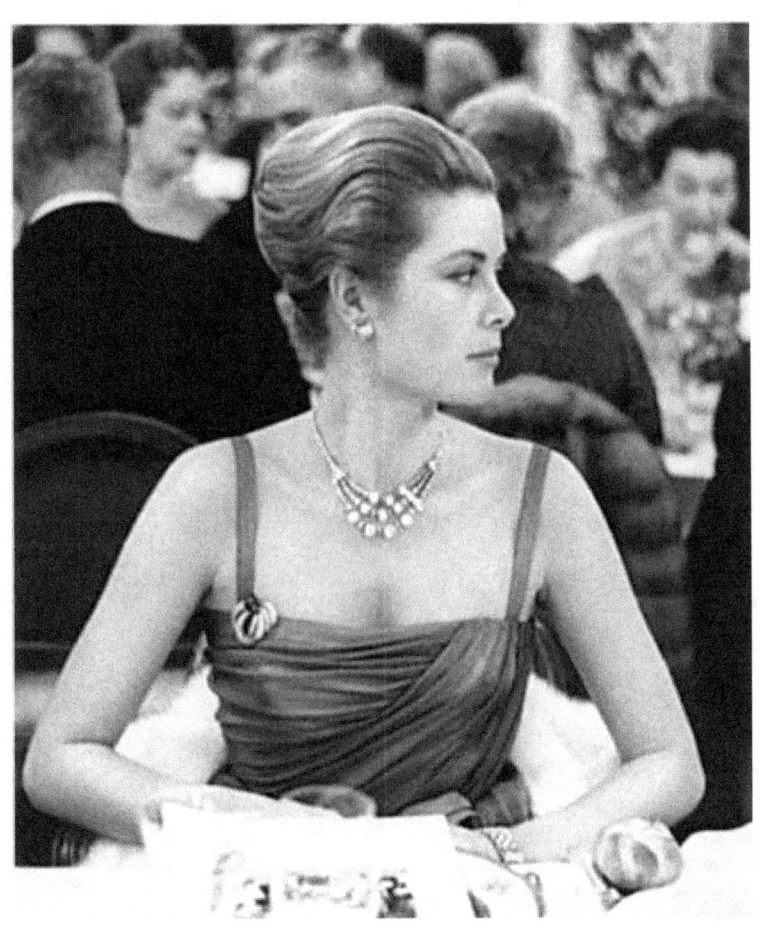

So if diva means giving your best, then yes, I guess I am a diva.
~ Patti LaBelle

My Story

I had let myself "go". I had some financial problems after a few layoffs during the Recession and wore the plainest "hand-me-downs" I found in churches and the Salvation Army. I was grateful for the discount clothing.

I was dating a very good-looking guy at the time. I was cutting my own hair to save $$. I was so dowdy, it was like I intentionally wanted to look plain.

Guess what happened? Another gal went after him. Her blonde tresses professionally streaked, her pretty clothes. She was fashionable. She looked great. And she knew how to flirt. Seductive? Oh yes. She greeted men "hi baby doll". She touched them, their arms, sometimes rubbed their shoulders.

 She pursued him relentlessly.

Well, the good news is, it was a temporary flirtation and ended quickly. He was too smart for her and saw through her shallowness. But it taught me a good lesson. I needed to change.

*"Never use the word "cheap".
Today everybody can look chic in inexpensive clothes
(the rich buy them too).
There is good clothing design
on every level today.
You can be the chicest thing in the world
in a T-shirt and jeans — it's up to you."*

~ Karl Lagerfeld

Princess Diana - a Transformation

In the early days Lady Diana was a frumpy dresser. She could look plain too.

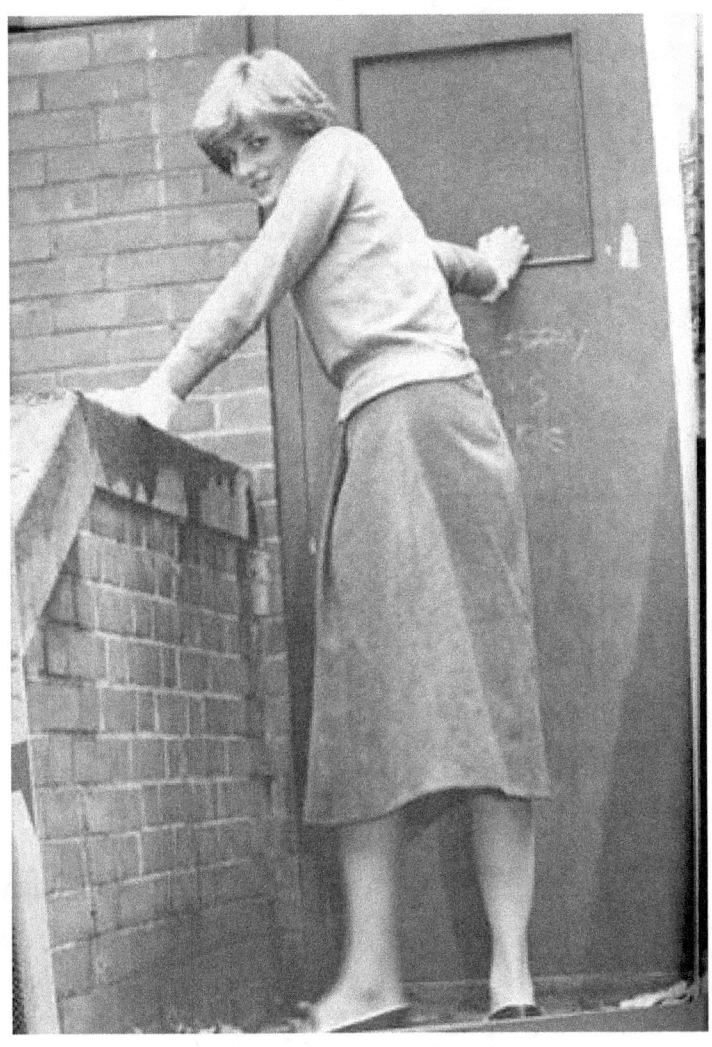

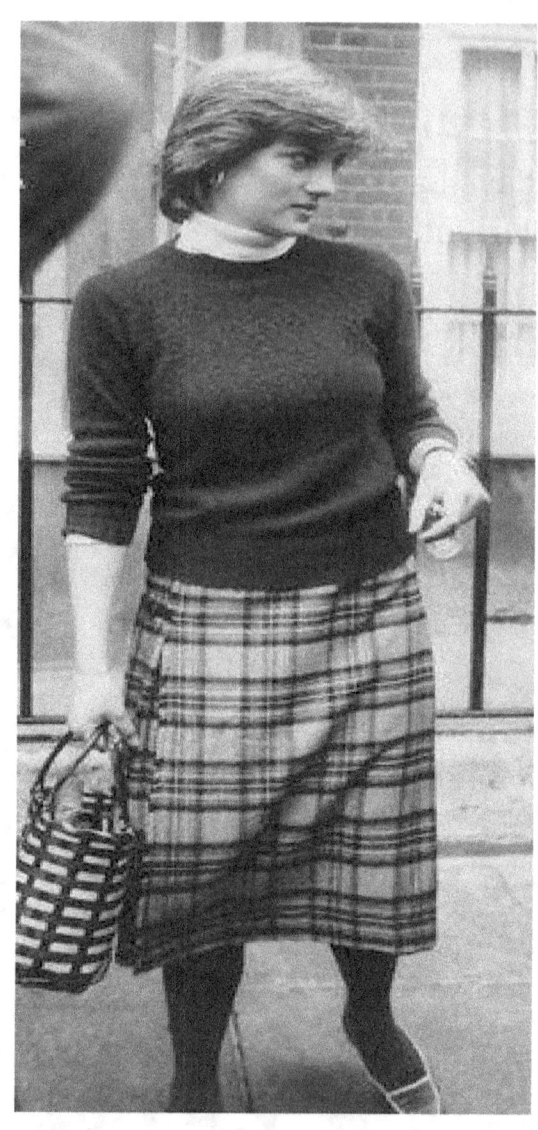

Look carefully at her clothes when she was "Lady Diana
Spencer". Not very eye catching. Blah. Plain. Not very
fashionable.

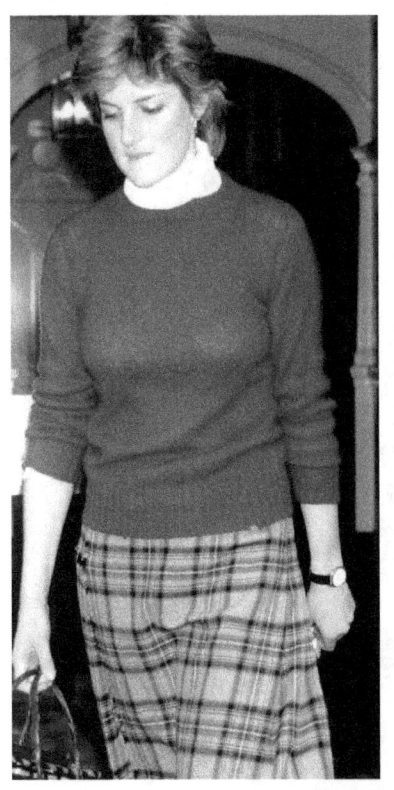
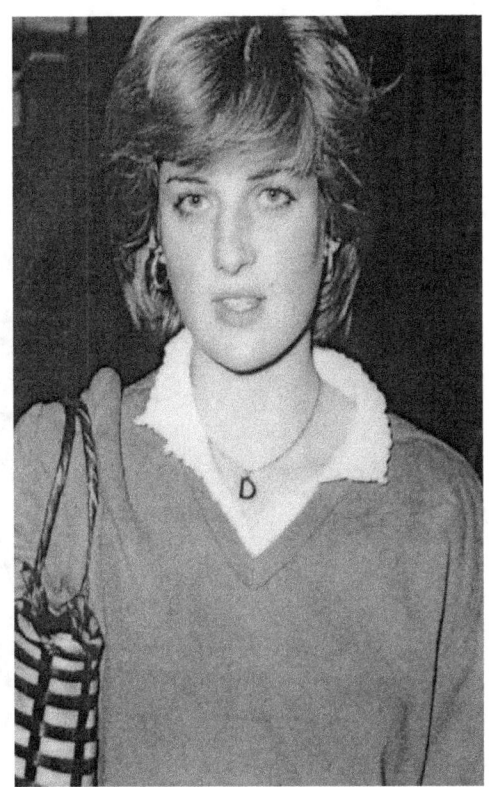
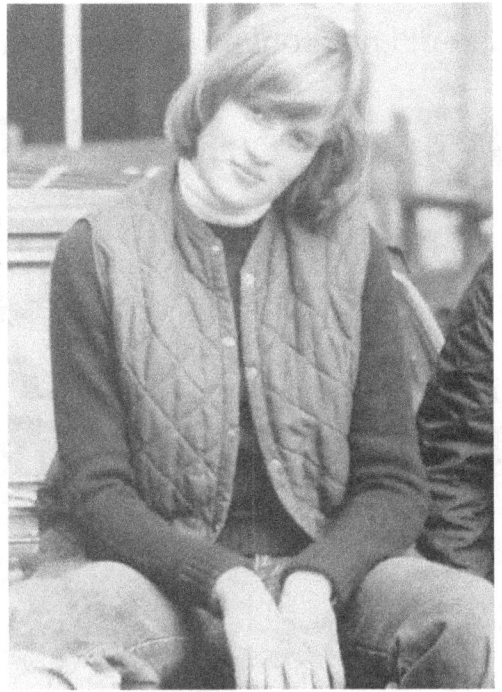

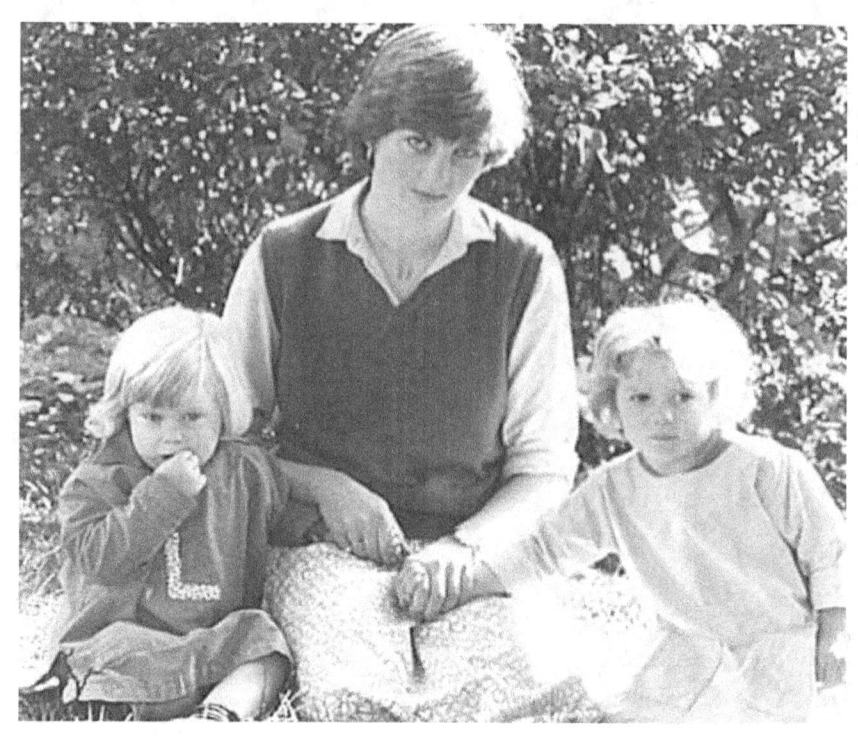

She did not convey self-confidence.

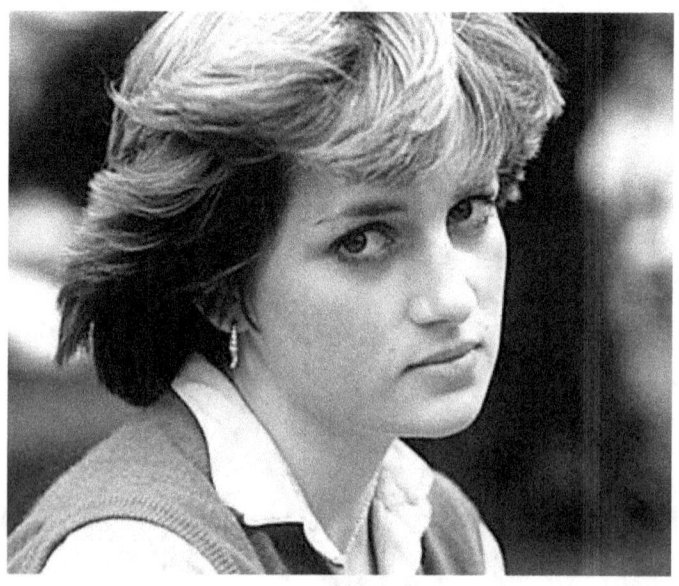

A "diamond in the rough".

Now watch her transformation:

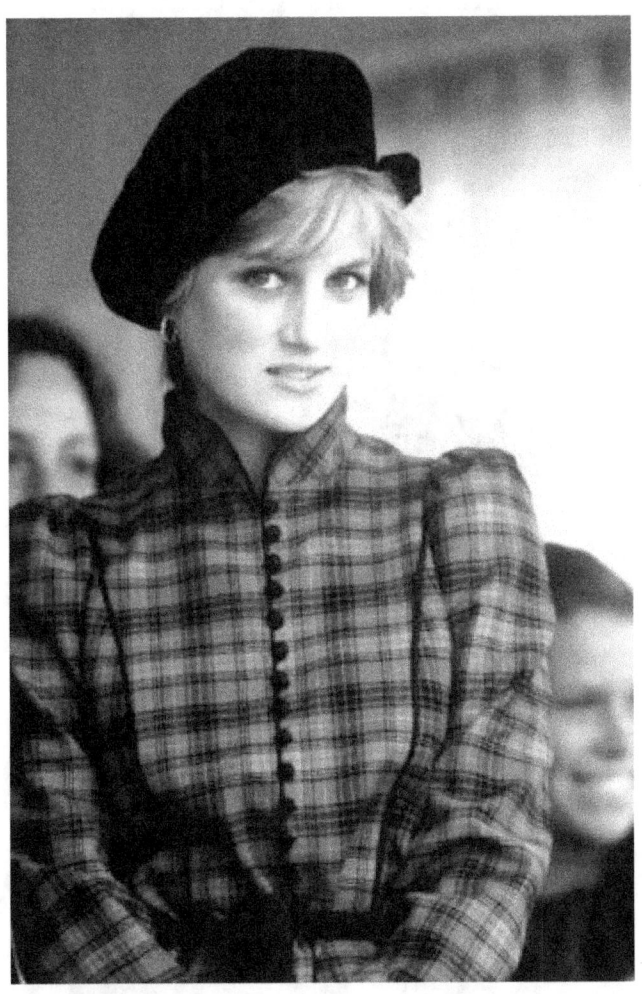

She lost the extra pounds:

\

Fashionable she became:

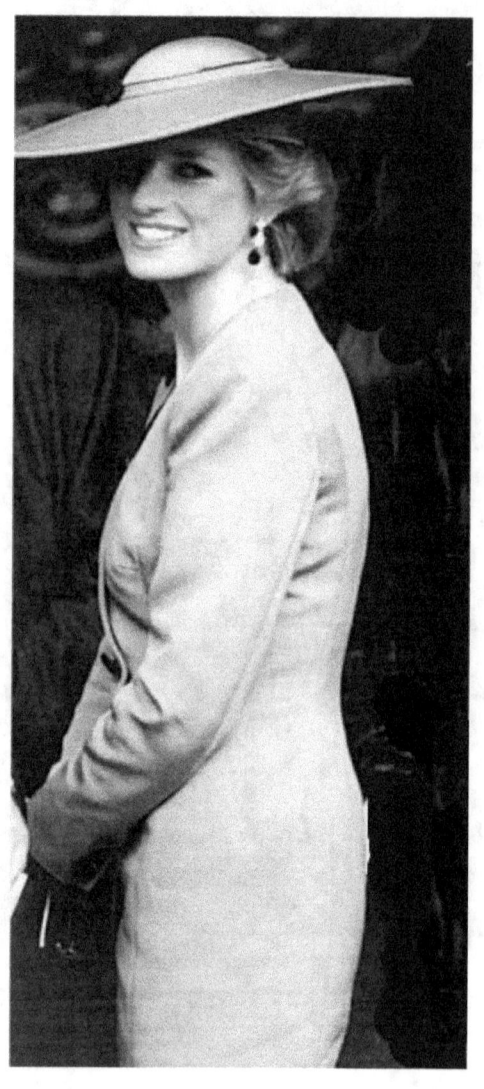

She was a smart girl.

She listened to her fashion advisers.

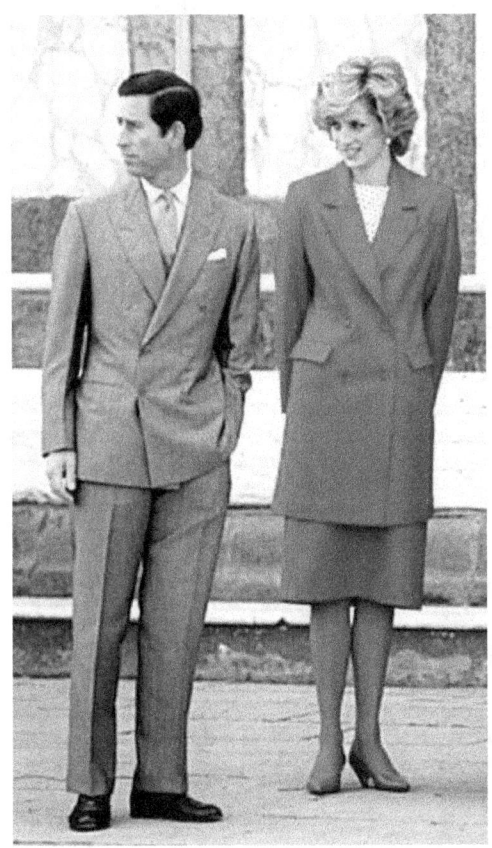 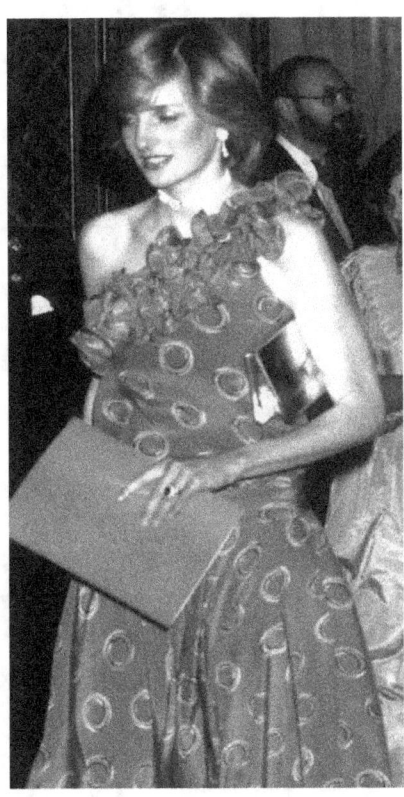

It takes a long time to get to be a diva.
I mean, you gotta work at it. ~ Diana Ross

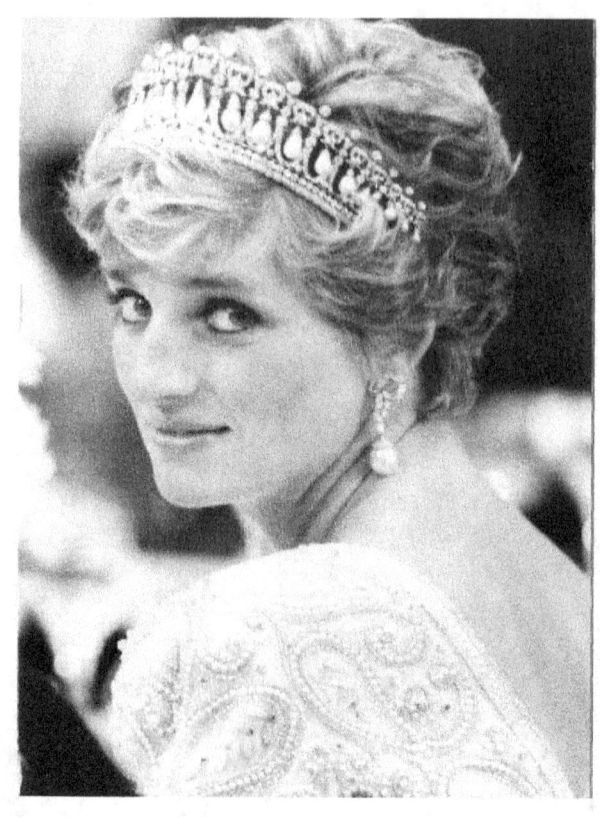

She became our beautiful Princess Di.

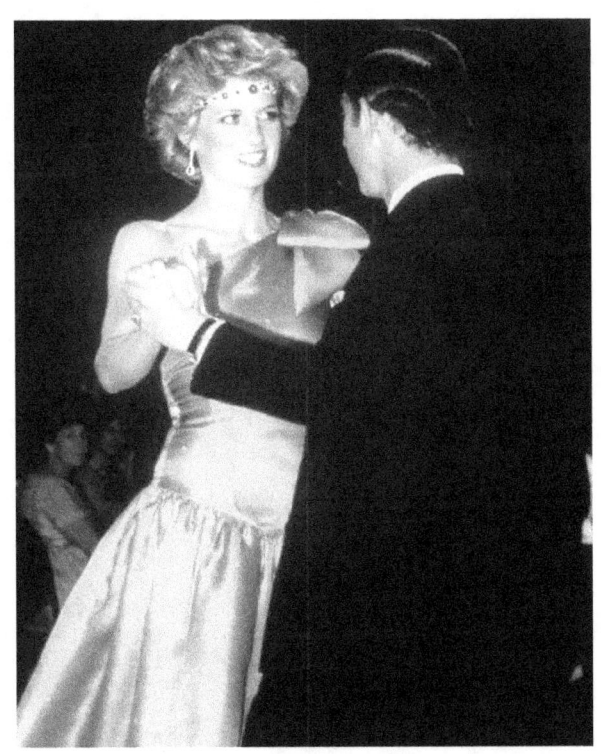

Beautiful inside and out...

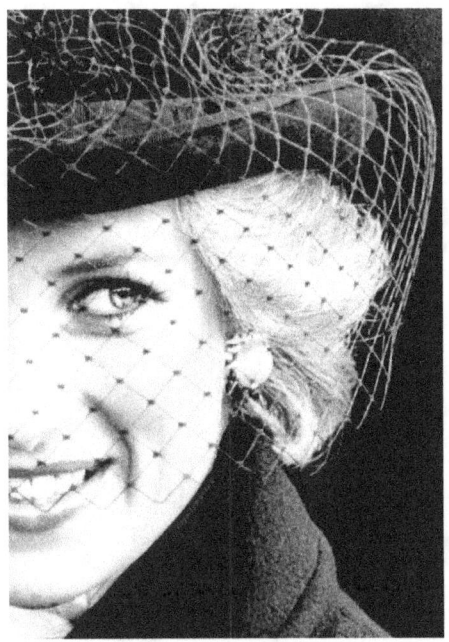

Style, What is it?

"You do not create a style. You work, and develop yourself; your style is an emanation from your own being."
~ Katherine Anne Porter

Style can be subtle. Simply a different texture can express style.

And you make style "your own". Become aware of what works for you. One person can carry off a certain style that makes you look silly, and vice versa.

People pay a lot of money for designer clothing. Why? Because it is "cut" well and hangs beautifully on the human body. Think about cut and fit, even if you purchase inexpensive clothes. Style is color, perceiving your body and personality and what works, cut and fit, fabric, etc. Everything comes into play. A small detail, a ruffle, a piece of lace, may express style. Grace Kelly had "it", Wallis Simpson did too.

Elegance

"Elegance is refusal." ~ Coco Chanel

Elegance has something to do with simplicity and restraint. A black dress is elegant. It is line and form and shape. We know it when we see it.

To me, I see a woman with elegance, who understands herself, who has given thought to design and fashion, and does not overdo it.

Dictionary Definitions:
- Refinement, grace, and beauty in movement, appearance, or manners.
- Tasteful opulence in form, decoration, or presentation.
- Restraint and grace of style.
- Scientific exactness and precision.

"The elegance is as physical, as moral quality that has nothing common with the clothing. You can see a countrywoman more elegant than one so called elegant woman."
~ Karl Lagerfeld

Clothes that "Fit"

"The human body is the best work of art."
~ Jess C. Scott

Some clothes are cut well and fit the curves of a woman's body to her advantage. Other clothes just hang loosely and make you look drab and dumpy. Why choose clothes that simply hang? We've all seen women who are dressed frumpily with nothing enhancing their look.

The feminine figure or shape is beautiful. Men respond to it. Let your clothes enhance your shape, without being brash about it.

Fit and cut are important!

Find clothes that emphasize your best attributes. If you have nice arms, go for a tank top, or if you want to show off your long legs, wear a short skirt.

I'm not a diva. I'm a tadpole trying to be a frog.
~ Toni Braxton

A Fit Body is a Style Statement

I spent years overweight. Let's face it: you are less sexy and attractive, some people will call you fat, people don't take you so seriously. Why go through life not at your best?

It doesn't matter what system you use, *but use something*!

If you are out of shape, perhaps start with Yoga. That how I started my fitness program.

What I Did:
I got serious. Eliminated sugar and bad carbs, bread, white pasta, white rice. Ate smaller portions.   Ate less cheese.

"No cookie is a good cookie" ~ Pete Abilla

Weight Watchers

The Weight Watchers Points System is a useful tool for those who want to lose or control weight. With this system, foods are assigned points. You count and control the total points of the food you take per day.

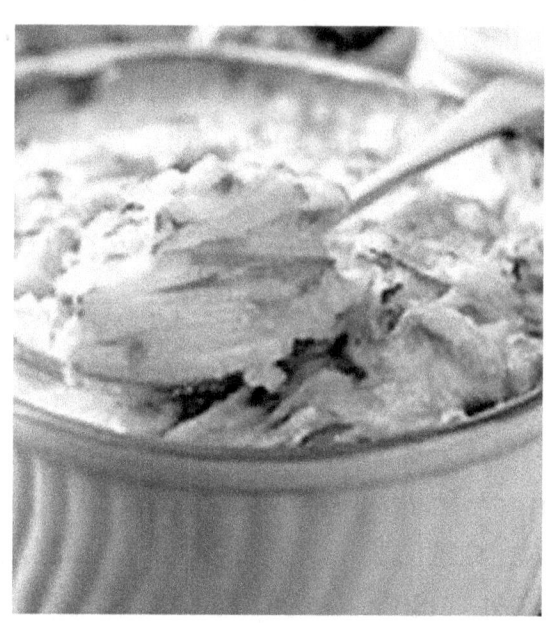

Au Gratin is Rotten!

At a church dinner, volunteers dished out 4 heaping cups of *au gratin potatoes* on my plate. I checked my Weight Watchers points book and saw that 1 cup was 12 points.

Well, my allowable points for the day were 25. If I ate 4 cups I would consume double my food allotment for the day! **No *au gratin* potatoes!** I ate the broccoli instead. You can eat unlimited broccoli and spinach -- these veggies have 0 points in Weight Watchers (Points Plus plan).

Weight Watchers has a new *PointsPlus* system. The new system is based on a formula of protein, carbohydrates, fat and fiber. It's a great food plan.

Fatties Cheat

We have all met the girls who know every diet, and rattle off the calories. But they are not losing weight. Why not? They cheat!

They scold you for using too much salad dressing. But how many "fatties" really get there from salads?? Let's get real.

I watched a very overweight acquaintance who whines about her weight, recently at a church dinner. I watched her a huge hunk of cornbread, then 3 desserts: apple pie with ice cream. Huh? Is she really serious?

It is time to get serious. This is your life. I became sick of being called "fat". I got serious. I went on a food plan.

I joined Overeaters Anonymous. I went on a food plan. I checked points in the Weight Watchers book. When hungry I snacked on 90 calories diet bars. AND IT WORKED!!!

I stopped eating any white pasta, processed bread, sugar, cakes, white rice. I reduced the amount of cheese I ate. My low carb diet worked for me. I lost 40 lbs.! This extreme diet may not be for everyone, but find one that works for you (please!!).

Example: A slice of pizza is 8 points in the Weight Watchers points book. I am allotted only 25 points daily. 3 slices of pizzas is almost my entire daily intake. Forget pizza! [maybe a slice once a month]. My diet was extreme, but my metabolism was as slow as a snail. There are many variations of food plans. Find one and stick to it.

Don't waste a minute not being happy.
If one window closes, run to the next window
or break down a door.
~ Brooke Shields

Movement
When you are more slender you move with grace. You become more attractive. You wear clothes better.

"A beautiful dress may look beautiful on a hanger,
but that means nothing.
It must be seen on the shoulders, with the
movement of the arms, the legs, and the waist."
~ Coco Chanel

I started dancing every Monday night. I started going to Jazzercise, a program of exercise through dance. Start a fitness program!

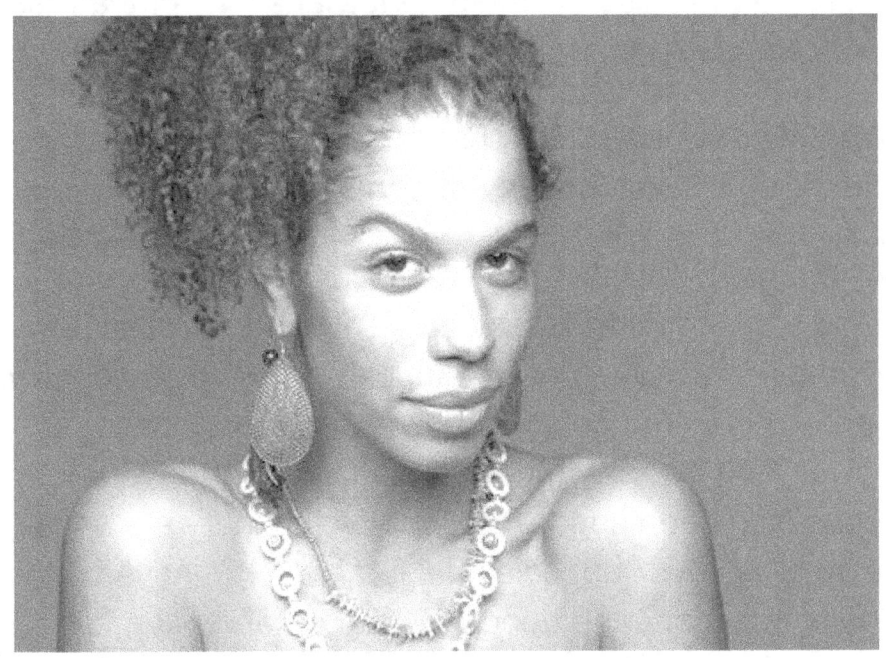

Diva has a negative connotation.
~ Glenn Close

Attitude

Women's Intuition

Women are generally recognized to have "intuition". Men have it too. But I see it more in women. It's a power we have, why not use it?

Many people said that Princess Diana had a gift of intuition. The first conversation she had with Princess Charles, she mentioned how sad he looked at the funeral of his beloved "uncle" Lord Mountbatten, how he needed someone to support him. At this point, Charles practically fell all over her, so much so, that Diana was embarrassed and confused.

What was the knack she had? She "felt" him, and perceived his real needs under his hard exterior.

Where does this ability to read emotions come from? It has been suggested that it is mainly due to social power. Women, who have been historically lower in social power, spend more time observing and scrutinizing those in power, and become more attuned to their nonverbal cues. It has also been suggested that evolutionary elements have been involved, selecting females who have better ability to decode the needs of children and potential mates. (*Psychology Today*, Ronald E Riggio Ph.D. on Jul 14, 2011)

> *"Fashion is not something that exists in dresses only. Fashion is in the sky, in the street, fashion has to do with ideas, the way we live, what is happening."*
> ~ Coco Chanel

Charisma

Have you ever met someone with charisma? They seem to have an energy, a light that shines.

Charisma is about creating rapport with people. It is not brash or overbearing either. *The Charisma Rules*, Gary Marshall

The term "charisma" has two senses: (1) compelling attractiveness or charm that can inspire devotion in others, (2) a divinely conferred power or talent.

Other definitions:
a special charm or appeal that causes people to feel attracted and excited by someone (such as a politician)

Since you are already (hopefully) enhancing your physical appearance, you have a glow. But a glow from inside also comes from a positive attitude, confidence, and caring for others.

Charm: the power or quality of giving delight or arousing admiration.

> *"I've learned that people will forget what you said, people will forget what you did, but people will never forget how you made them feel."*
> ~ poet Maya Angelou

Presence
I know a woman who walks around slouched over, dragging behind her a backpack on wheels. She looks sad and self-absorbed. Do you want to be around her? No!

Being in love with life, or acting cheerful attracts people to you.

"And now, I'm just trying to change the world,
one sequin at a time."
~ Lady Gaga

Seduction

Seduction is not cheap or vulgar. Seduction is something that attracts or charms. It's a hint, a mere taste, an appetizer. It can be elegant.

It may be a glance. Letting a man know you find him pleasing, attractive. Not every man or woman is talented in this area. Watching films and actors can be instructive.

Be sophisticated, not trashy.
Intelligence is seductive. Don't suppress your values and morals. Be you.

Do not lay everything on the table. Always reveal things slowly to him. Find your own style here.

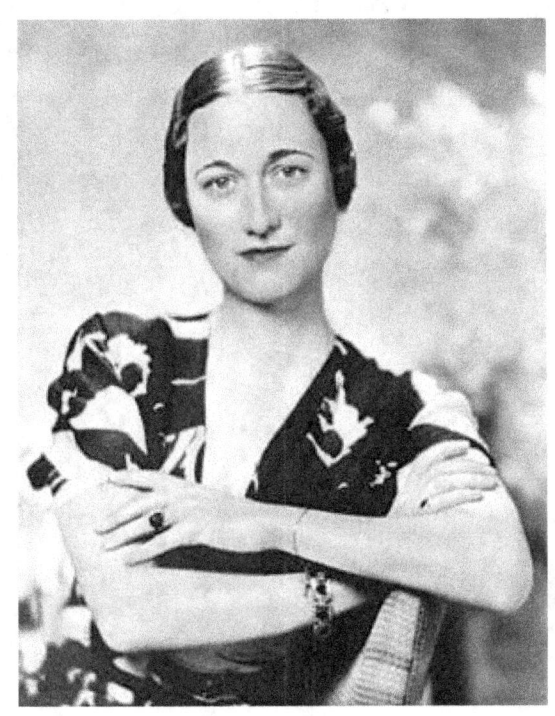

Wallis Simpson - Seduction

Wallis Simpson, (the Duchess of Windsor) knew the art of seduction well.

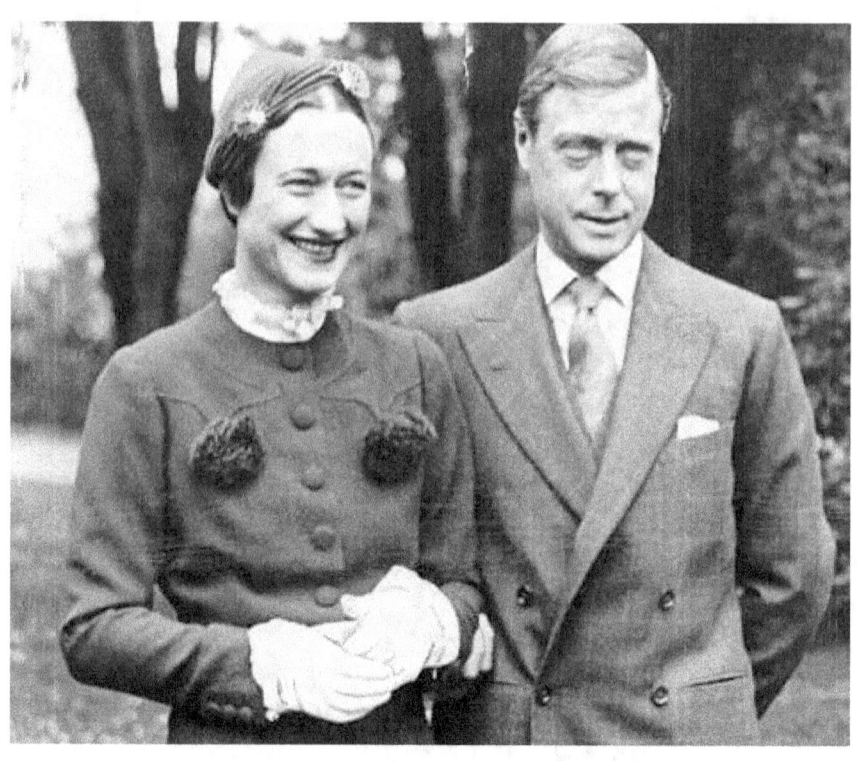

Wallis Simpson, married Prince Edward, Duke of Windsor, formerly King Edward VIII, who abdicated his throne to marry her. It was her third marriage. It was the scandal of the century.

She appeared to have a magnetic power to attract men. Many who knew her have commented on her sex appeal, her contagious laugh and — in the words of a friend — 'beautiful dark sapphire blue eyes, full of sparkle and nice mischief'. (Read more: Daily Mail)

Wallis' father died when she was five months old and she and her mother had to rely on irregular handouts from a wealthy relative. Born Bessie Wallis, she had ditched the first part of her name as fit only for cows and, according to one of her friends, brazenly announced that she wanted to marry for 'lots of money'.

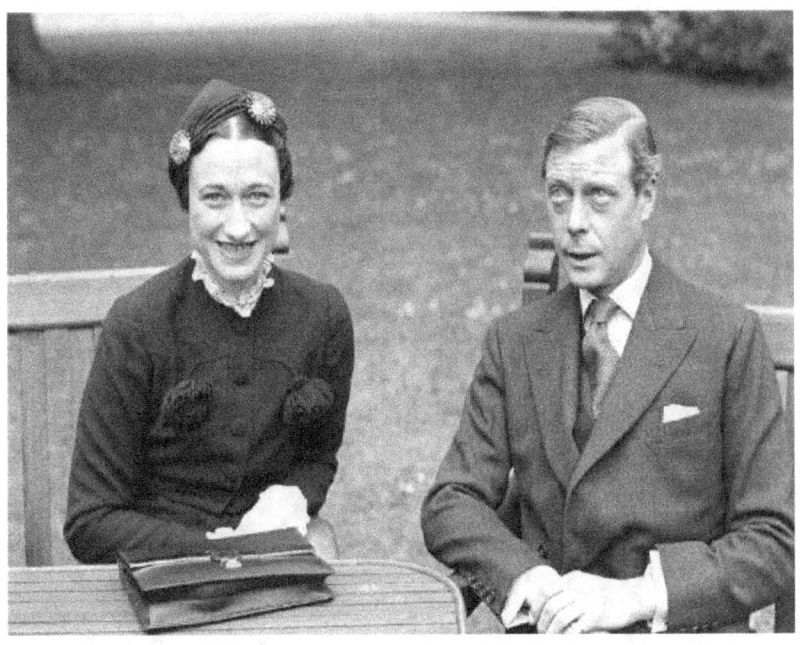

Wallis realized she wasn't a great beauty but stated she had decided to be thinner and more fashionable than others. And she was!

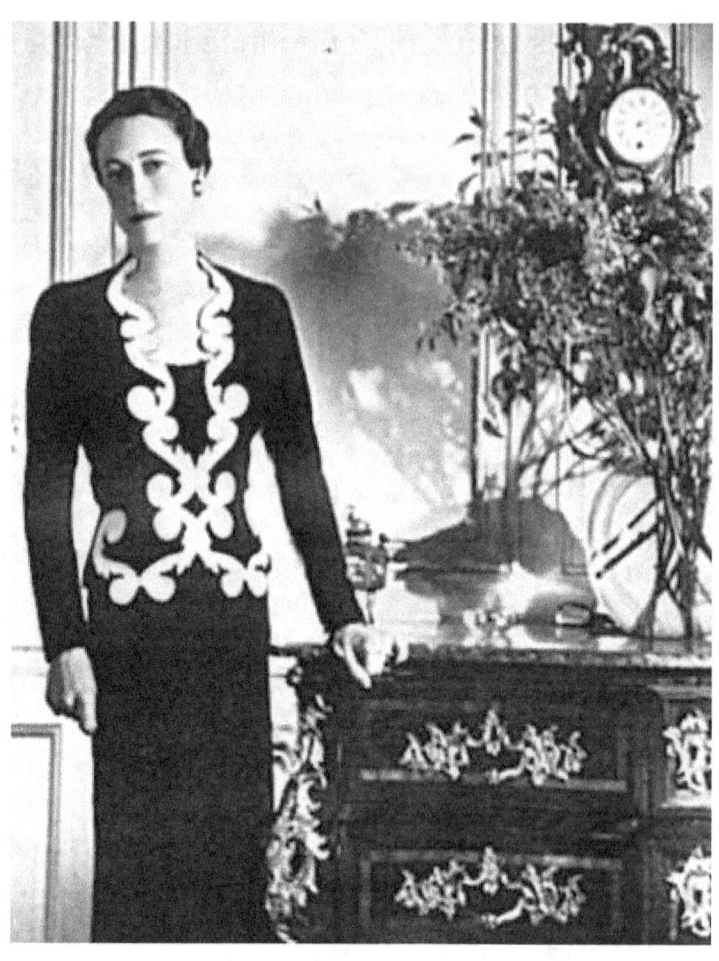

She had an incredible style sense and wardrobe.

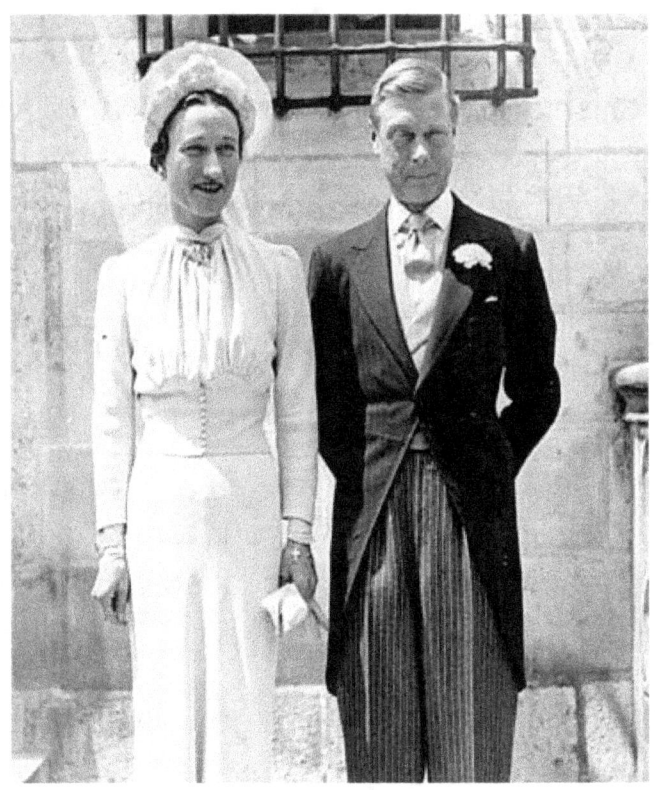

She won her Prince.

We don't have many descriptions about Cleopatra, but one thing for sure, Marc Anthony rearranged his entire life for her, left his wife. She is described as a beauty.

Spend time pondering what seduction is.

Here is a great Youtube video talk by Dr. Seema Anand, "The Art of Seduction":
https://www.youtube.com/watch?v=jnS66SszwEs

Dealing with Male Attention

An extra cushion of fat will keep men "at a distance", and there are times we use it. It's unconscious probably, a way to avoid men and sex and relationships.

In my first meeting of Overeaters Anonymous we talked about how we had used extra fat to avoid the arena of sexuality.

Lose the weight, get fit and you WILL receive more male attention. It is inevitable. And you Deal With It! Some men you want to "cool down" because you are not interested, plain and simple.

This is a real issue that will emerge. You are no longer invisible.

Flirting

Light flirting. It really is so easy. I used to be so frightened of flirting. How silly. It's just light attention and friendliness toward someone. It can be fun. It doesn't have to mean much, just letting someone know they are attractive to you. It's a compliment. I used to be so serious about it, like asking a man for coffee was so important. I would ponder, "will he make a good father?". Silly…. It's just coffee!!!!

But flirting may also be an avenue to meet a mate, so it can be serious too. Practice it.

Make the first move occasionally.

"Even the manliest of men don't like to face rejection and get their feelings hurt. We're probably all for trying to pick you up, but give us a hint that we may have a shot before we dive in. If you're not going to initiate an interaction then maybe open your body posture, touch us on the arm, or shoot us a warm smile — just give us an excuse, any excuse, to think we won't be humiliated if we make a move, and we'll be happy to strike up a conversation. "(*13 Things Men Think About Women But Never Say,* Cody Delistraty)

A compliment (or two) doesn't hurt. Men are insecure too.

As you talk to a man, establish eye contact. Make your eyes expressive. Let your eyes talk. Give him a captivating glance and try to express what you really want using your eyes. Make him notice that you are actually flirting so that he won't get the wrong signal.

Men are Visual

Remember men are visual. Use that piece of knowledge. Look a little sexy or at least sensual. Play with it. It's fun.

I see men as honey bees and women as the flowers. Bees seek the prettiest, most fragrant flowers. Same with men.

Men struggle with visual temptation

This means the vast majority of men respond to visual images when it comes to women. And, this doesn't just mean the guys with wandering eyes. Even a good husband cannot avoid noticing a woman who dresses in a way that draws attention to her body. Even if it is just a glance, these visual images are stored away in the male brain as a sort of "visual rolodex"; that will reappear without any warning. Men can choose whether to dwell on these images and memories or dismiss them, but they can't control when these images appear. (source: _For Women Only: What You Need to Know About the Inner Lives of Men_, Shaunti Feldhahn)

Allure and Mystique

"The most beautiful makeup of a woman is passion. But cosmetics are easier to buy."
~ Yves Saint-Laurent

Carolyn Bessette Kennedy - Effortful Effortless

Another style Queen, God rest her soul, who married John F. Kennedy Jr.

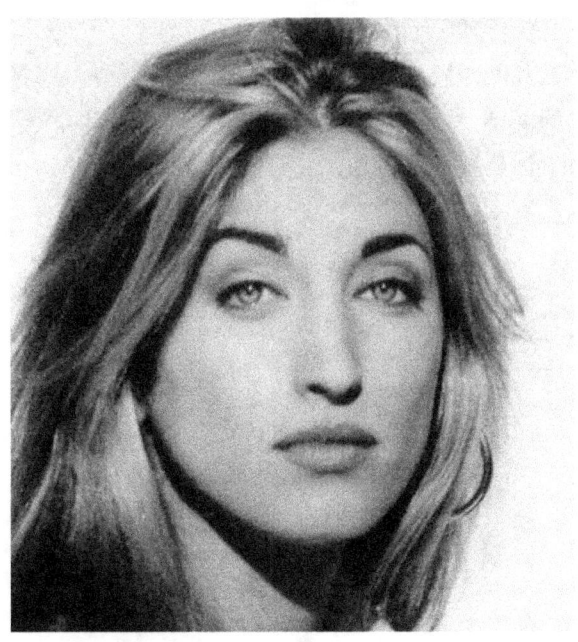

Caroline Bessette landed a job at a Calvin Klein store in Boston, reportedly hired by a boss who spotted her walking down the street. When she actually met Klein, the fashion designer was so impressed that she was transferred to the New York headquarters.

"She knows how to handle men like practically nobody I've ever met," a friend of Kennedy, John Perry Barlow, told New York magazine. "She is very good at making people feel they are special and important, and largely because she means it."

Caroline's style was described as "throwaway chic" and "effortful effortless." But don't kid yourself, there was a lot of effort involved.

Carolyn was always beautiful BUT these in early photos we see a plainer Carolyn, before she discovered the fashion world, before finding her own style.

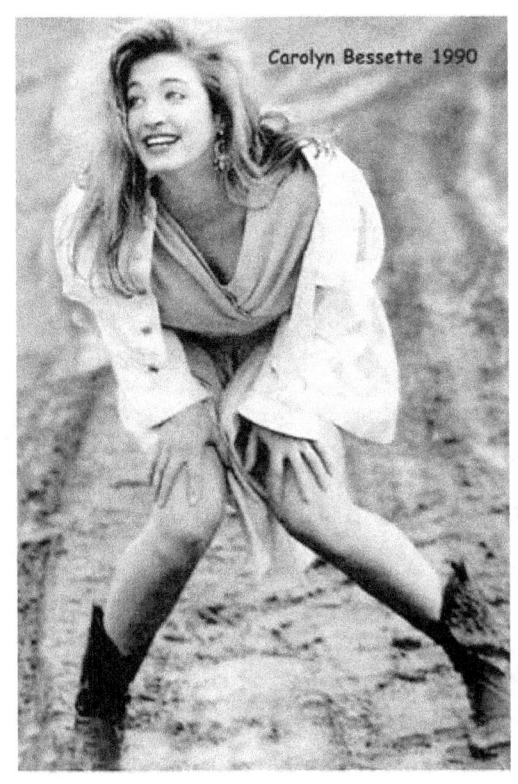

Carolyn Bessette 1990

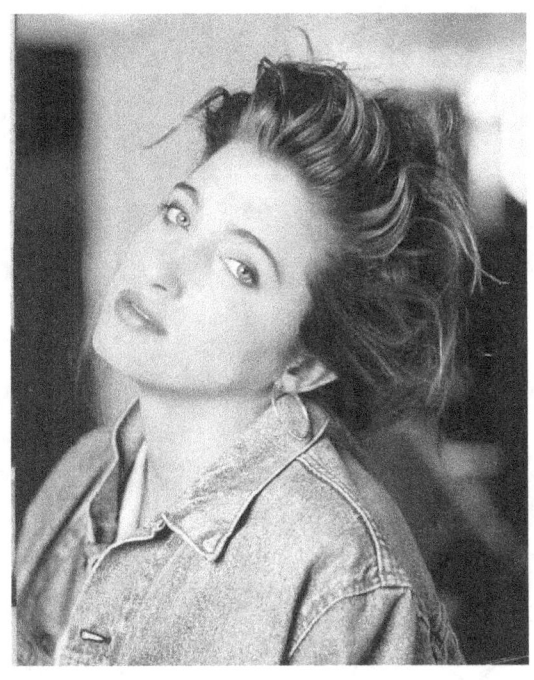

A much plainer Carolyn:

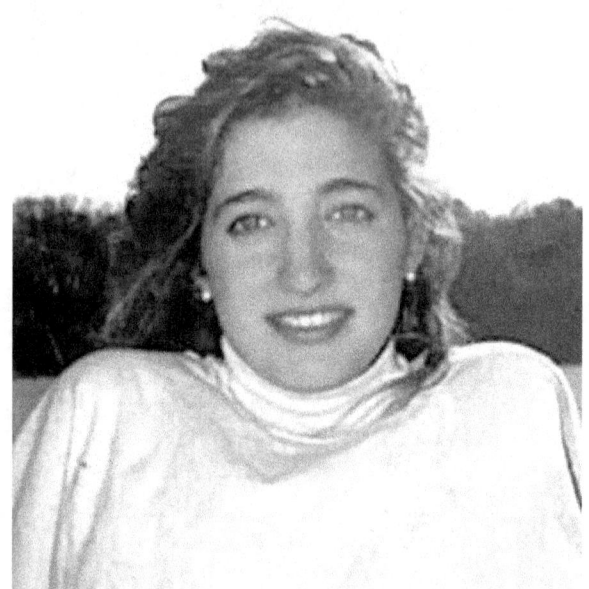

Carolyn was drawn to the fashion world. She learned fashion, hairstyles, and make-up, evolving into a stunning woman.

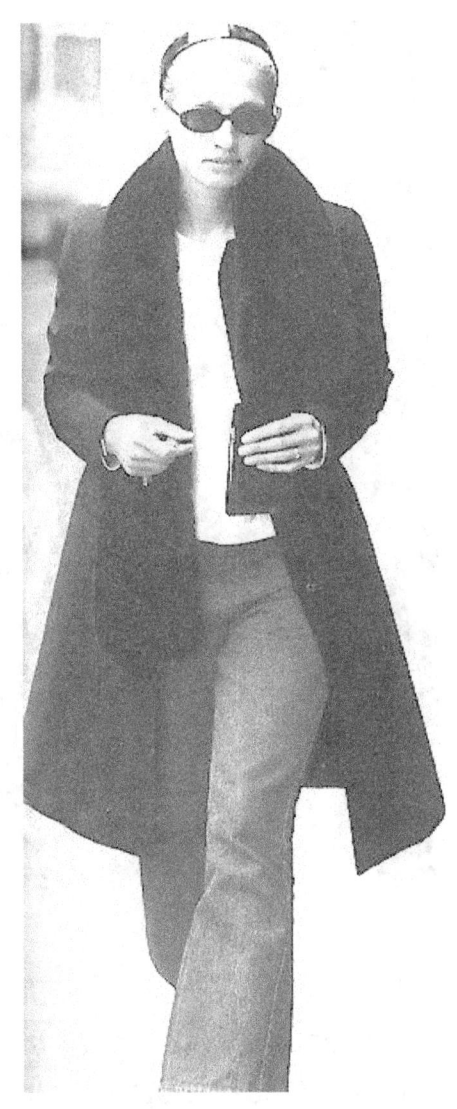

"Black is modest and arrogant at the same time. Black is lazy and easy - but mysterious. But above all black says this: "I don't bother you - don't bother me"."
~ Yohji Yamamoto

Look at the lines of the dresses below; just beautiful.

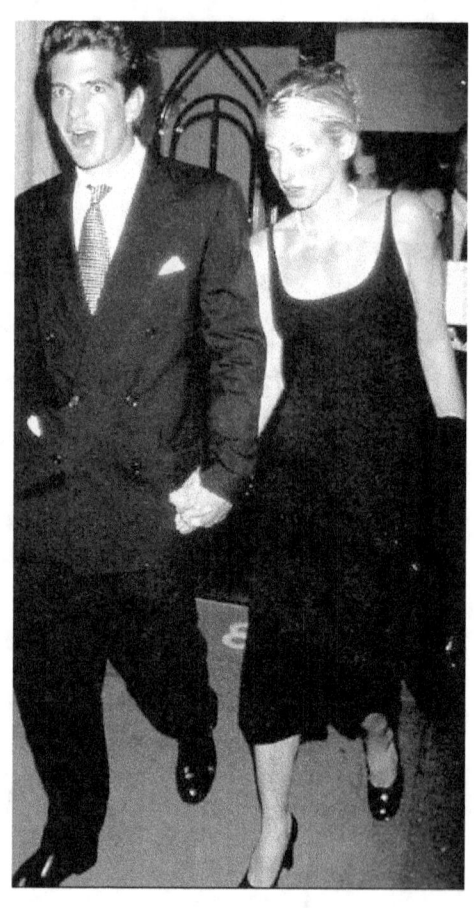

"She was wearing a purple T-shirt, with a skinny black dress over it that made you remember how much of a girl she was, and trashed black boots that made you forget."
~ Kami Garcia, *Beautiful Creatures*

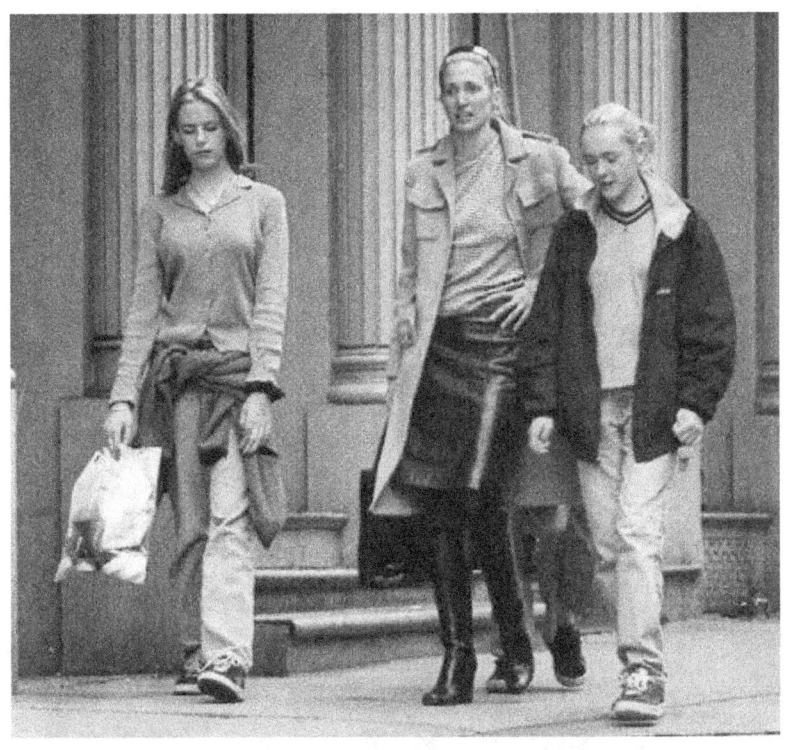

And who could forget her wedding gown?

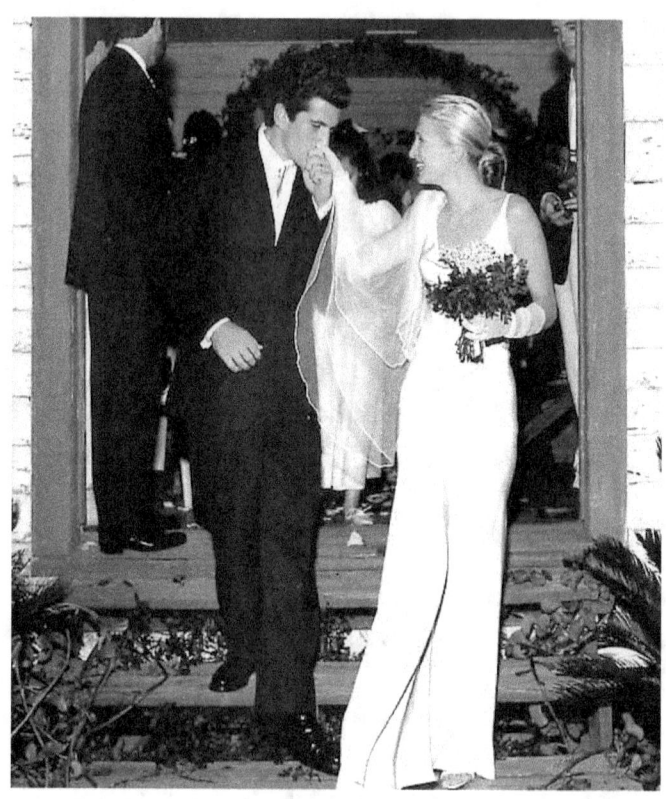

Another woman, who skillfully learned to let her beauty shine.

More Beauty Tips:

Skin

Use exfoliating creams or masques. Some have fine particles that scrub away the old cells and bring a radiance to your skin. I started using one and people told me "you have a glow". And I did.

Hair

Do some investigation on how to improve your hair. I used henna on my hair, and it brought highlights and improved texture to my hair.

You Are Already Beautiful

When all is said and done. We are all beautiful already. Without make-up. Just being born, what a miracle.

And personality and confidence make a woman physically sexier. But what is wrong with enhancing this beauty??

And beauty is in the eye of the beholder. I loved my dog who was a mutt, but she was a beauty to me. Gorgeous.

On YouTube there is a great video by model Cameron Russell where she talks about being beautiful and how women need to strive for more than mere looks: " Looks Aren't Everything. Believe me, I'm a Model."
https://www.youtube.com/watch?v=KM4Xe6Dlp0Y

Looks are not everything, but this book was about enhancing you. Become your most beautiful you. Let the world see your brilliant light. Tell the world, with your clothing, your movements, your fit beautiful self that you ARE beautiful!

Actually, I take it as a compliment. Diva is a derivative of divine. That's quite a title to carry around. ~

Calista Flockhart

More Resources:

YouTube Videos:

"How to stop screwing yourself over" by Mel Robbins
TEDxSF
https://www.youtube.com/watch?v=Lp7E973zozc

contact: safeinthewoods@gmail.com

www.ingramcontent.com/pod-product-compliance
Lightning Source LLC
Chambersburg PA
CBHW070820290526
45795CB00002B/782